Allergy, Toxins,

and the

Learning-Disabled Child

George von Hilsheimer

Superintendent, Green Valley, Florida,
a special residential school for
children and adolescents with
learning disabilities.

Academic Therapy Publications
San Rafael, California

1974

Acknowledgements

The author gratefully acknowledges the valuable contributions made by L. S. Moore and T. Tucker in the writing of the section entitled "Minor Physical Abnormalities in LD, BD, and ED Children."

Special thanks and appreciation are due to E. L. Binkley, MD, and S. Klotz, MD, for their advice and encouragement, which helped this work to become a reality.

7721/

International Standard Book Number: 0-87879-078-0

Library of Congress Catalog Card Number: 74-75287

Printed in the United States of America.

Contents

5   Allergy, Toxins, and the
     Learning-Disabled Child

31   Screening for Allergies

47   Notes On Nutrition

51   Minor Physical Abnormalities
     in LD, BD, BD, and ED Children

61   Recommended Reading

63   Photographic Essay of Genetic Signs

Allergy, Toxins and the Learning-Disabled Child

In 1965 we recruited, at Green Valley, a vivacious young woman as a technician in our neurophysiology and behavior modification lab. Although she had no college training she had been on the staff of the marine biology lab of a major university as a mass spectrometrist and micropaleontologist. She was a very intelligent, popular, outgoing, well organized, and competent person, capable of an enormous amount of skilled work.

Several months after joining us, Mrs. Black became very irritable. She began to have serious marital problems. She became less competent at work. From having been the center of social activity, her office became a solitary cell. She began to choose very dark, often black clothing. She painted her bedroom dead black (enough of a reason for marital conflict). She painted her office dead black.

I began to think of Mrs. Black in psychodynamic terms. "She cannot accept the pressure of responsibility in a novel community that does not use time clocks and other management devices." "She cannot adapt to the importance of her husband's role in our program." "She has always controlled the society around her; and her habitual methods don't work in this therapeutic environment; therefore she is attempting to control by being sick."

Mrs. Black became increasingly fatigued, tense, antisocial, and incompetent. (She had spells when she could not type, and temporary periods when she could not read.) My response was exasperation—after all, I knew she had greater capacity than she was presently demonstrating; and this childish retreat was not worthy of such a gifted person.

It occurred that a hemophyliac student had a crisis and blood was needed. A number of staff went down to give blood. The nurses could not locate any blood pressure on Mrs. Black. This fact managed to penetrate even *my* prejudiced head, and we rushed her to our internist, Dr. Sol Klotz.

After a thorough workup Mrs. Black was returned to us with a diagnosis of food allergy—pork and tomatoes being the prime villians. This was really too much for me. I called Dr. Klotz and said, "Sol, you have to be kidding. I mean, there has to be something *wrong* with her." You will notice, of course, that my brilliance neglected to illuminate the fact that an allergy might be something profoundly wrong. After all, everyone *knows* allergies are psychosomatic.

Sol and I have worked together for many years, and he tolerates my presumptions. He patiently instructed me on the importance of taking him seriously, mildly inquired if I had a diagnosis I would like to substitute; and we closed the issue. Pork and tomatoes were removed from her diet. In about six weeks Mrs. Black was again vivacious, fully alert, competent, a social butterfly, full of energy and enthusiasm. Her husband seemed somewhat bewildered by the rapid change, but the marriage had obviously been set abubble with life again.

It took this event to force me to begin to take my own scientific value system seriously. For several years Dr. Klotz had been serving as primary care physician for Green Valley's adolescent students when they became ill. In those days we initially relied on the referring doctor's examination and history. (We no longer do.) The children who were sent to Dr. Klotz for a variety of ills frequently returned with a diagnosis of allergy, and with prescriptions and routines for their treatment. Since I had a great deal of respect for Dr. Klotz, both as a person and a physician, I did not allow my exasperation with his "fixation" to dissuade me from using him as our primary care physician; however, I was often heard to mutter, "Well, an allergist just has to diagnose allergies."

Imagine! Over the course of years a physician whom I respected and trusted had returned a very high percentage of students to us after careful evaluation with a diagnosis of allergy. Rather than being compelled by the evidence, I was snared in a psychodynamic prejudice and so, for years, ignored hard facts.

6

After the episode involving Mrs. Black, we began to send students randomly to Dr. Klotz for allergy screening. The percentage of allergic students, often with no allergy reported in their histories, was extremely high. This information was intriguing; however, we remained suspicious of the extremely high percentage. We began to screen all of our children for allergies.

In November 1972 Dr. Klotz reported that 103 of 107 sequentially admitted students had proven to be significantly sensitive to at least three of twelve allergens tested.[1] These tests were conducted in a double-blind fashion—the students did not know which injections were allergens and which placebo, nor did the physician reading the initial response, nor the nurses reading the delayed response.

The accumulation of data over the years has convinced us that a major factor in the disturbance of learning skills in children is an allergic reaction to ordinary substances, and especially to food.

A large majority of the children sent to us, particularly the boys, are physically immature. This finding is widely reported in the literature of exceptionality. D. Sandberg has reported that a survey of 100 growth-retarded children indicated a great increase in growth when highly allergenic foods, such as wheat, corn, and milk, were removed from their diet.[2]

Sandberg has more recently reported in great detail on the precise effects of food allergy on growth in height of children.[3] He has found that, when these children are removed from the foods to which they are sensitive, that the growth curve normalizes but there is no "catch-up" growth.

"Catch-up" growth is a well documented finding. Children restored to normal diet after severe malnutrition, or taken off steroid drugs, or otherwise treated so that the growth curve normalizes, experience a spurt of accelerated growth and usually catch up with their age peers. The food-allergic child apparently merely normalizes his growth curve, but remains behind his age peer norm for actual height. However, Sandberg has found that if these children receive hypodesensitization injections (very dilute preparations of food extract) the "catch-up" growth spurt occurs. Sandberg has demonstrated that growth is exquisitely sensitive to allergic stress. The growth curves plotted for his subjects show an almost immediate response to eating allergenic foods, to their removal, and to treatment or lack of treatment with hypodesensitization injections. He chose growth as his measure because it is perhaps the most objective measure that can be made in children.

P. J. Collipp reported that the asthmatic child and those who suffer from eczema are frequently developmentally immature.[4] His center is coordinating a national study of the use of pyridoxine with these children (who also show poor tryptophan metabolism and almost certainly suffer food allergies and intolerances).

Edward L. Binkley, Jr., MD, brought our attention to the fact that a sequence of minor physical traits we had seen in our children has been reported in the literature and is seen in his practice of allergy, which specializes in hyperkinetic and learning-disabled children.

Binkley's list of traits includes very fair complexion, electric hair, a double crown in the hair, epicanthal folds, low set ears, adherent earlobes, malformed ears, soft and pliable ears, high steepled palate, furrowed tongue, geographic tongue, curved fifth finger, single transverse palmar crease (Down's line, or the Mongoloid line), third toe longer than the second, partial fusing of the middle toes, and a gap between the first and second toes.[5] Similar information has been reported by M. F. Waldrop and C. F. Halverson, Jr., and J. L. Rapoport, P. O. Quinn, and F. Lamprecht, for hyperkinetic children.[6]

Our own list is considerably larger and was influenced by J. W. Tintera's report of characteristic physical traits in patients with insufficient adrenal-cortical function and resulting low blood sugar.[7] (See pages 51-60 for the full list of minor physical anomalies associated with systemic disease, learning, behavior, and emotional disabilities.)

These physical traits are seen in hyperkinetic children significantly more often than in normal children. They are seen in boys more often than in girls. They are often associated with a wide range of symptoms (fatigue, faintness, chills, tension, and the like).

We have surveyed populations in California, Texas, Florida, and New York; and we have found that (of our entire list) the normal population averages about three of these traits. Hyperkinetic, learning-disabled, and behaviorally disordered children average about seven, and psychotic or severely emotionally ill children average about thirteen. These results are highly significant.

The distribution of these traits among these populations is quite distinctive. The control populations fall in a normal bell-shaped curve. This indicates that the usual random influence of genetic distribution occurs to produce the traits in a control population. The treatment groups fall into an approximately equal distribution. In other words, about the same number of children have five, six, seven, eight, or more signs to the top of the range. This produces a flat line indicating that a strong non-random factor is influencing the ordinary genetic selection. (See Distribution of Physical Traits, page 10.)

The discovery that our students have a significantly higher number of distinctive physical anomalies lends support to other findings we have reported. Since 1968 we have monitored every student on a wide range of biochemical assays. These assays also demonstrate that our group is significantly different from controls.

Ninety-nine percent of entering students do not demonstrate any spillage of free ascorbic acid on admission. More than 80 percent do not demonstrate any spillage after loading with three grams of ascorbic acid per day for two weeks.

Almost no child admitted to our center demonstrates metabolic balance or efficiency. Over 90 percent are deficient in manganese. Almost all are severely depleted in tissue potassium and sodium. Many are deficient in iron and zinc, and most are toxically high in copper and lead. Eighty-six percent demonstrate irregularities in glucose and insulin metabolism. About 25 percent demonstrate extremes in values of serum fats. Other indications of deficiencies, of malabsorption of food, and of poisoning, are often found.

Leon Rosenberg has reported on a number of gene-linked vitamin-dependency diseases discovered in the last decade.[8] In these disorders the body cannot metabolize ordinary foods efficiently, and must receive enormous multiples of vitamins.

If the urine demonstrates high values of homocystine, a metabolic product of tryptophan (an essential amino acid), it is clear that the body does not normally utilize pyridoxine (vitamin B-6) and therefore cannot metabolize tryptophan but produces poisons. Children with this disorder are frequently diagnosed as autistic. Treatment for several months with 400 mg of pyridoxine a day enables the child to function normally. This supplementation must continue the rest of the child's life. It is not a question of a vitamin deficiency, not an inadequate diet, but a *dependency*. The individual cannot efficiently handle the chemical and depends on an enormous quantity to be able normally to function.

DISTRIBUTION OF PHYSICAL TRAITS

```
0
1   xxxxx
2   xxxxxxxxxx
3   xxxxxxxxxxxxx
4   xxxxxxxxx
5   xxx
6   x                    Control Group
7   x
8   x                    N=42   Mean=3.14   Median=3   Mode=3


0
1   x
2   xx
3   xx
4   xxxx
5   xxx
6   xxxx
7   xxxx
8   xx
9   xx
10  xxxx
11  xx               Learning-Disabled Group
12  xxx
13  xxx              N=36   Mean=7.36   Median=6   No Mode


0
1
2
3
4
5
6   xx
7   x
8   xx
9   x
10  xxx
11  xxxx
12  xxx
13  xxxx
14  xxxx
15  xxxxx
16  xxxx
17  xxxx
18  xxx          Severely Emotionally Disturbed Group
19  xx
20  xxx          N=48   Mean=12.66   Median=14.5
21  xx
22  x            No Mode
```

10

CONTINUOUS BOY–GIRL GROWTH CHART

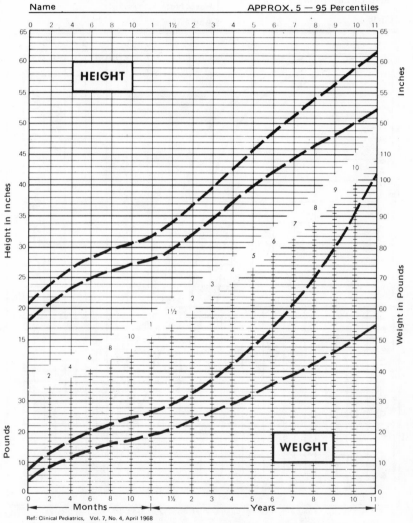

Name _____   APPROX. 5 — 95 Percentiles

HEIGHT

WEIGHT

Height in Inches

Pounds

Inches

Weight in Pounds

Months —— Years

Ref: Clinical Pediatrics, Vol. 7, No. 4, April 1968

Distributed as a Service by Mead Johnson Laboratories, Evansville, Indiana 47721

Lit. 257, 11/69

11

Head Circumference Chart
Girls

HEAD CIRCUMFERENCE
GIRLS

+2SD (98%)

mean (50%)

−2SD (2%)

MONTHS

YEARS

CM

IN

Ref:Nellhaus,G.,Composite International & Interracial Graphs,PEDIATRICS 41:106,1968.
University of Colorado Medical Center Book Store

Head Circumference Chart

Boys   SIDE FOR GIRLS)

Date

Ward

Name

Hosp. No.

Address

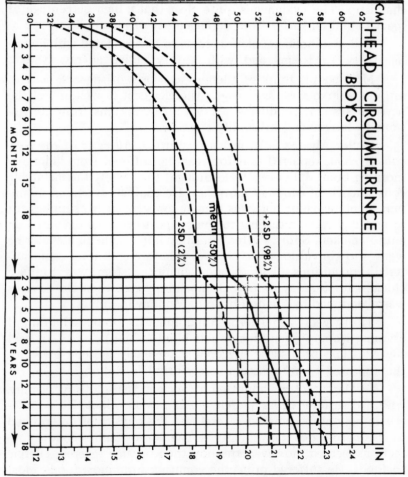

Ref:Nellhaus,G.,Composite International & Interracial Graphs,PEDIATRICS 41:106,1968.
University of Colorado Medical Center Book Store

13

Collipp and his colleagues have found other metabolites of tryptophan, kynurenine and xanthurenic acid, are frequently high in immature, allergic, asthmatic, and eczematous children.[9] Again, treatment with pyridoxine (which is the coenzyme enabling efficient tryptophan metabolism) permits normal functioning.

We now routinely study all of our children for the metabolites of vitamins, as well as protein, fat, glucose, and insulin chemistry. The evidence is quite clear that a high percentage of special children suffer from derangement of metabolism.

This metabolic imbalance seems to be associated with hypersensitivity to toxins and with a very active allergy system.

Most people think of allergies as causes of sneezes, coughs, asthma, skin rashes, and hives. Allergies can, as well, affect the nervous system, producing a range of symptoms from convulsions to fatigue and irritability.[10]

Walter Alvarez, MD, in his forward to *Allergies of the Nervous System*, reported that for years he suffered from "Monday morning brain dullness."[11] He thought this merely the inevitable consequence of Monday mornings. He took an extended mountain climbing jaunt and was caught away from his supplies for several days. On returning to the support cabin he devoured an entire chicken. Shortly after returning home some hours later he went into convulsions. He had never before and never again suffered convulsions. The Alvarez family custom was to have chicken for Sunday dinner. On abandoning chicken Dr. Alvarez was abandoned by the dull brain of Monday mornings.

Thirty years ago Theron Randolph, MD, presented a film of a young woman given (in a double-blind fashion) placebo or beet sugar.[12] The beet sugar triggered a three-day episode in which she appeared to be in a completely drunken state.

In May 1971 we admitted a fourteen-year-old boy, Dennis, who had suffered from allergic eczema as an infant. His secondary infections became so severe that the physicians determined to use heroic doses of cortisone. The eczema and secondary infections cleared; however, the boy then became severely allergic to foods. He suffered projectile vomiting from most foods. Most of us know that projectile vomiting is a symptom of serious brain tumor; however, most allergists know it as a symptom of severe food allergy. It does not seem too great a leap to suggest that the brain may directly be involved in these allergies. Dennis' mother had been told that he would be a dependent adult, that there was nothing that could be done for him. In his thirteenth year he

14

gained but two pounds and was severely emaciated. His diet had been so restricted that his teeth had only two points of bite and were very irregular and poorly formed. He was quite cooperative with his diet, since the results of violation were so dramatic and rapid.

After verifying that severe food allergies continued to afflict Dennis, and having discovered no foods which did not provoke a severe skin reaction, we placed him on a hypodesensitization routine. He was also moved in with a staff family with only one other foster child, a nonverbal girl, and four natural siblings. Dennis was given freshly juiced organically raised vegetables in small quantities to build up his vitamin and mineral balance, and slowly to decondition his fear of eating. He was also given vitamin supplements specially prepared to avoid allergens.

In six weeks we began feeding small amounts of normal foods on a rotary basis. No food was repeated more than once a week.

By December we were prepared to discharge Dennis, who was able to visit his family for Christmas. We retained him until May to complete remedial education and to follow up preparations for orthodontal reconstruction.

During the spring Dennis developed upper-respiratory-tract (URT) symptoms, sniffles, and sinusitis. Placing a highly efficient air filter in his bedroom relieved the symptoms. When the filters were removed without his knowledge the symptoms returned. Subsequent use of the filter fully reduced the URT symptoms.

Dennis returned home in May and was enrolled in the tenth grade in a private school for ordinary children. (He had been regarded as a retarded failure in the seventh grade when sent to us the previous year.)

Dennis' shift of allergies from one system of the body to another was not unusual. First his skin was affected, then his gastrointestinal tract and brain, and then the URT. It has long been noted that schizophrenics almost never suffer URT symptoms, until they are cured or in remission. It would seem that strong symptoms in one body system tend to prevent symptoms in another. Since the brain is a large and sensitive organ, its immunity from allergic reactions would be remarkable. This is particularly true since we know that both toxins and allergic reactions can cause a great increase in intracranial pressure.[13] Cerebroasthenia, or brain exhaustion, caused by infection, trauma, toxin, malnutrition, stress, and allergy, is well established as a source of deranged learning and behavior.[14]

Assessing these children, we find there is a high correlation between severity of symptoms and the physical traits reported by Binkley, Tintera, Waldrop, and Green Valley. When evaluating adult control groups, we find that about 75 percent who report five or more of the physical traits have a serious systemic disorder—asthma, diabetes, atherosclerosis, hypothyroidism, etc. When we evaluate the remaining 25 percent, we find that they often do not see physicians regularly but do have symptoms; and many of them are obese. We regard plus 10 percent overweight as a systemic disorder. Most physicians agree with us.

It is quite clear that learning disabilities, behavior disorders, and emotional disturbances are not isolated entities but exist in a complex matrix with metabolic efficiency of the body and the occurance of systemic disease.

Assessing the Child

If a child displays the following attributes, we can be pretty certain we will also see a child who is hyperkinetic, immature, and showing the signs of minimal brain dysfunction:

- fair-haired (much fairer than either parent),
- fine, light hair which drifts or stands out,
- "orientalish" pouches over his eyes,
- frequent bags, or shiners, or dark rings under the eyes,
- irregular teeth, or missing, or extra teeth,
- a high-steepled palate,
- index finger is longer than his ring finger,
- only one line across his palm (one that is either straight across or stops, and does not curve up between the index and middle finger),
- a big gap between his great and second toes (and the third toe is as long as the second or longer).

Say he is eight years old and has difficulty walking a straight line, especially on tip-toe, or on his heels, or backwards. He cannot stand still with his eyes closed and hold his hands straight out, palms flat, but tends to raise them up or lurch. If we ask him to hold his hands out and copy us while we match our right thumb to each of the fingers, he will likely have mirror movements in his left hand—even if we bring his attention to the fact that we are not moving our left hand at all. He is not likely to be able to touch our moving index finger with his index finger while alternately touching his nose. Often he will report only one finger touching him when we are touching two places on his back, and will have difficulty "reading" a letter we draw firmly on his back with our finger. He will almost certainly have reading problems. (Hyperkinetic Checklists for parents and teachers are on pages 19, 20, 21, and 22.)

This child will also almost surely have perceptual problems. On a test of reaction time he will probably be deviantly fast or progressively slower. If he is fast, he will become faster as he becomes more tired, or the longer we test. He will have many false starts. If asked to press a button for a rose light but not for a red, he will rapidly be unable to do the task properly. If we increase the rate and shorten the length of the signals, he will have difficulty. If we ask him to press a bulb strongly for the rose light and weakly for the red, he will homogenize the presses as the task is made more difficult. The same will occur for a red light/green light, or for long-tone/short-tone signals. If he is a slow responder he will soon not respond at all.

This boy will almost certainly be an allergic child; his glucose metabolism very likely will be deviant; and he will have about a 25 percent chance of having a deviant protein, fat, insulin, or thyroid metabolism. He will almost certainly spill no ascorbic acid in his urine, regardless of his diet; and he will very likely have metabolites of amino acids or enzymes in his urine which reflect dependencies and inefficient metabolism. If he has every one of these traits, symptoms, signs, and deficiencies, we may see a very sick child indeed who has been diagnosed as schizophrenic, autistic, or psychopathic; but, in some cases, he may simply be regarded as a head-strong boy, difficult to discipline, who just doesn't like school. "But he is really so bright, and so good with his hands, and just charming when he wants to be and a terrific athlete." Or, "He never gives us any trouble, but he can be so stubborn, and he just can't stand school, they just don't understand him."

It is almost certain that his mother has been told:

• there is nothing wrong with him;

• boys are slower than girls;

• he will outgrow it;

• you are just overanxious and making him worse; or,

• he is extremely emotionally ill, and you must have the whole family in for regular psychotherapy.

These comments will have been made despite the fact that other children in the family are quite competent, well behaved, excellent scholars. The response to this is, "You are scapegoating this child." The assumption that parents, particularly mothers, are incompetent and overanxious appears to be thoroughly trained into all too many doctors in their first year of schooling.

It has been well established that the mothers of children with severe crippling disease, diseases with high rates of mortality risk (osteporosis, tuberculosis, diabetes, asthma) and other severe chronic diseases behave very much like the mothers of schizophrenics and other emotionally ill children. The child disturbs the family. Removal of the child from the family is often followed by a dramatic improvement in the relations of the whole family. The terrible reality of severe diseases and strong behaviors cannot be ignored even by superparents.

Psychic Energizers

Frequently such children respond to psychic energizers. They almost never respond to barbiturates or tranquilizers, although these are often prescribed.

One three-year-old was seen by me at his parent's home. Henry was extremely fair, had epicanthal folds, his index finger was longer than his ring finger, his teeth were somewhat irregular, his third toe was longer than his second, and he had a large gap between his great and second toe. He had not slept a full night in his life, was extremely hyperactive, could pull himself from the crib at age ten months, ran at eleven months, and went frequently into paroxysms of rage and terror. His mother was fatigued but very patient. His one-year-old sister was a model of cuddly sweetness and security.

At my suggestion his parents requested the pediatrician to attempt Dexedrine or Ritalin. He would not, saying these are dangerous drugs, even though he had the boy on phenobarbitol—which made his behavior worse. (Phenobarbitol is a sedative or hypnotic. The child is anesthetized, and the brain does not go through the normal ninety-minute cycle when barbiturates and other "sleeping pills" are used. Dream-time and the deepest stages of sleep are suppressed; therefore, the child is not rested. A similar situation occurs when adults drink too much, "sleep" suddenly, and are exhausted the next day. Unconsciousness is not sleep.) The parents persisted in seeking a physician who does his homework and found a doctor who prescribed Dexedrine (dextroamphetamine). The boy's behavior normalized. In about six months Dexedrine lost its effectiveness and Ritalin (methylphenidate) was prescribed. Henry remained on Ritalin until his

PARENT'S QUESTIONNAIRE

CAUTION: The SAME parent must perform
all evaluations.

Name of Child _____

Date of Evaluation _____

INSTRUCTIONS:
- Answer ALL questions: examples are given to clarify some.
- Your first rating is meant to give a pre-treatment standard of comparison with other children the same age.
- Subsequent ratings should compare the child's behavior and attitudes NOW against your FIRST rating.

Beside each item below, indicate the degree of the problem by a check mark (√) meaning . . .	Not At All	Just A Little	Pretty Much	Very Much
1. Picks at things (nails, fingers, hair, clothing).				
2. Sassy to grownups.				
3. Problems with making or keeping friends.				
4. Excitable, impulsive.				
5. Wants to run things.				
6. Sucks or chews (thumb; clothing; blankets).				
7. Cries easily or often.				
8. Carries a chip on his shoulder.				
9. Daydreams.				
10. Difficulty in learning.				
11. Restless in the "squirmy" sense.				
12. Fearful (of new situations; new people or places; going to school).				
13. Restless, always up and on the go.				
14. Destructive.				
15. Tells lies or stories that aren't true.				
16. Shy.				
17. Gets into more trouble than others same age.				
18. Speaks differently from others same age (baby talk; stuttering; hard to understand).				
19. Denies mistakes or blames others.				
20. Quarrelsome.				
21. Pouts and sulks.				
22. Steals.				
23. Disobedient or obeys but resentfully.				
24. Worries more than others (about being alone; illness or death).				

(Over)

19

	Not At All	Just A Little	Pretty Much	Very Much
25. Fails to finish things.				
26. Feelings easily hurt.				
27. Bullies others.				
28. Unable to stop a repetitive activity.				
29. Cruel.				
30. Childish or immature (wants help he shouldn't need; clings; needs constant reassurance).				
31. Distractibility or attention span a problem.				
32. Headaches.				
33. Mood changes quickly and drastically.				
34. Doesn't like or doesn't follow rules or restrictions.				
35. Fights constantly.				
36. Doesn't get along well with brothers or sisters.				
37. Easily frustrated in efforts.				
38. Disturbs other children.				
39. Basically an unhappy child.				
40. Problems with eating (poor appetite; up between bites).				
41. Stomach-aches.				
42. Problems with sleep (can't fall asleep; up too early; up in the night).				
43. Other aches and pains.				
44. Vomiting or nausea.				
45. Feels cheated in family circle.				
46. Boasts and brags.				
47. Lets self be pushed around.				
48. Bowel problems (frequently loose; irregular habits; constipation).				

49. If there are any additional comments on these questions or any remarks not covered—please elaborate below.

_____

_____

50. If this is the *first* rating form you have completed for your child, answer the question marked 50A. If not the *first* rating, answer question 50B.

  (50A) How would you rate your child compared to other children the same age?

  ☐ Much Worse ☐ Worse ☐ About the Same ☐ Better ☐ Much Better

  (50B) How would you rate your child NOW compared to your initial evaluation?

  ☐ Much Worse ☐ Worse ☐ About the Same ☐ Better ☐ Much Better

_____
Signature

_____   _____
Relationship to Child   *Date Completed*

20

TEACHER'S QUESTIONNAIRE

CAUTION: The SAME teacher must complete
all evaluations.

Name of Child _____

Grade _____ Date of Evaluation _____

INSTRUCTIONS:

- Answer ALL questions: examples are given to clarify some.
- Your first rating is meant to give a pre-treatment standard of comparison with other children the same age.
- Subsequent ratings should compare the child's behavior and attitudes NOW against your FIRST rating.

Beside **each** *item below, indicate the degree of the problem by a check mark (✓) meaning . . .*	*Not At All*	*Just A Little*	*Pretty Much*	*Very Much*
1. Restless in the "squirmy" sense.				
2. Makes inappropriate noises when when he shouldn't.				
3. Demands must be met immediately.				
4. Acts "smart" (impudent or sassy).				
5. Temper outbursts and unpredictable behavior.				
6. Overly sensitive to criticism.				
7. Distractibility or attention span a problem.				
8. Disturbs other children.				
9. Daydreams.				
10. Pouts and sulks.				
11. Mood changes quickly and drastically.				
12. Quarrelsome.				
13. Submissive attitude toward authority.				
14. Restless, always "up and on the go."				
15. Excitable, impulsive.				
16. Excessive demands for teacher's attention.				
17. Appears to be unaccepted by group.				
18. Appears to be easily led by other children.				
19. No sense of fair play.				
20. Appears to lack leadership.				
21. Fails to finish things that he starts.				

(Over)

	Not At All	Just A Little	Pretty Much	Very Much
22. Childish and immature.				
23. Denies mistakes or blames others.				
24. Does not get along well with other children.				
25. Uncooperative with classmates.				
26. Easily frustrated in efforts.				
27. Uncooperative with teacher.				
28. Difficulty in learning.				

29. If this is the *first* rating form you have completed for this child, answer the question marked 29A. If not the *first* rating, answer question 29B.

   (29A) How would you rate this child compared to other children the same age?

   ☐ Much Worse   ☐ Worse   ☐ About the Same   ☐ Better   ☐ Much Better

   (29B) How would you rate this child NOW compared to your initial evaluation?

   ☐ Much Worse   ☐ Worse   ☐ About the Same   ☐ Better   ☐ Much Better

30. Please add any information concerning the child or his home and family relationships which might have bearing on his behavior.

_____

_____

_____

_____

_____

_____

_____

_____

_____

_____

_____

_____

_____

_____

_____

_____

Signature

Title   *Date Completed*

seventh year. He is a precocious youngster, an excellent reader and chess player since his fourth year. He has mild allergies, obviously with central-nervous-system involvement, a prediabetic glucose curve, and now can be maintained on nutritional supplements only. He does regress to hyperkinetic behavior or rages when extremely fatigued or frustrated. This case tends to support the cerebroasthenic theory of hyperkinesis.

Other Biological Disorders

It is important that parents not stop working on the problem if symptoms are relieved by Ritalin, Deaner, Dexedrine, or other energizers. All such children should be worked up for allergies, should have sugar taken as thoroughly out of their lives as possible, and should be evaluated for thyroid imbalance. As they reach adolescence their fat and insulin metabolism should be evaluated. Their urine should be tested at least twice a year, particularly after loading the night before with a rich meal high in sweets. If sugar or acetone is produced, a physician should order a study of blood glucose and insulin.

Let me emphasize that many children have been sent to us after years of "medical" treatment during which diabetes has been missed. This is outrageous, but not uncommon. Far too many psychiatrists and psychiatric hospitals do not insure that their patients be treated by primary care physicians. (See Biochemical Checklist, page 24.)

Frequent Disorders

About 25 percent of our students demonstrate very unusual fat metabolism. No one who has followed the autopsy reports from the Korean and Viet Nam wars or from auto accidents should be surprised. Fatty deterioration and blockage of the arteries and heart has been found to a surprising degree in young people. In a significant number of our students the ratio of phospholipids to cholesterol is quite high (norm: 1.0 to 1.2; our exceptions as high as 3.0). These fats are lost through toxic or allergic reactions in the central nervous system since the two primary phospholipids are constituents of the nervous system only. Other students show clear evidence of genetic predisposition to the various types of atherosclerosis and diabetes.

About 15 percent of our students demonstrate hypothyroidism. The chronic low production of thyroid is often a factor in mental illness. Full-blown symptoms of the cretin con-

BIOCHEMICAL CHECKLIST

Blood Assays

Complete Blood Count (CBC)

VDRL

Calcium
Inorganic Phosphatase
Glucose
Blood Urea Nitrogen
Uric Acid
Cholestrol
Total Protein
Albumin
Bilirubin
Alkaline Phosphatase
LDH and SGOT
Triglycerides
Phospholipids
Insulin
Galactose
NAD
B-12
Folic Acid
T-4 (Murphy-Pattee Method), and T-3
Thyroxin

Urine Assays

Random Van der Kamps (for ascorbic acid)
Random Acetone
Random Sugars

Creatinine
Thiamin (B-1)
Riboflavin (B-2)
Niacin (B-3)
Pantothenic Acid (B-5)
Pyridoxine (B-6)
Estrogens
Testosterone
17 Ketosteroids
17 OH Steroids
Cortisol
Diagnex Blue
Schillings Test (when indicated)

dition, or myxedemic madness, need not be present. Low normal or low thyroid findings in individuals with learning, behavior, and emotional symptoms, particularly those with pallor but no anemia, lethargy, edema or puffiness, and poor attention indicates to our physicians that thyroid supplement should be tried.

Evidence of inefficient absorption is clear in more than half of our students. Parasites cannot be ruled out in children from middle- or upper-socioeconomic backgrounds. This is particularly true for adolescents—in whom they are seldom sought. Worms are frequently found in adolescents who have adopted the hippy style.

Most of our students demonstrate some degree of vitamin deficiency or dependency. All learning-disabled children are under stress. All stress accelerates the need for nutriments. All stress decreases efficiency of absorption and metabolism.

Bernard Rimland, MD, reported a survey of 1591 emotionally ill children treated by drugs and found 27.7 percent helped, but 26.7 made worse. The best drug, Mellaril, helped 36.4 percent and made 19.9 percent worse. In this group he found 191 children who had been treated with high doses of vitamins; 66.5 percent were improved and only 3.7 were made worse by vitamin therapy.[15]

Vitamin B-12 and folate anemias are surprisingly common among our children, and our consultant staff find that the frequency of these deficiencies among their adult patients is even higher.

Many of our adolescents produce insufficient growth- and sex-hormones. These hormones have multiple functions and must be balanced if maximum restoration is to be enjoyed.

Metal Metabolism

A very large number of our children have a high value of lead in their tissues, even though our norms are adjusted by recent studies of human hair from 1875 to 1925, in which lead values were ten times those of contemporary hair. Blood and urine tests are not adequate measures. Lead can be stored in fat and tissue to be released later. Often a child will present symptoms during periods of heat or strong physical exercise, or on drug treatment for some other disease. Some drugs, heat, exercise, or weight loss will cause fatty tissue to give up stored lead, causing irregular appearance of symptoms. We believe a tissue biopsy is important. Fortunately, the literature indicates that hair is an adequate material for analysis.

Our hair analyses have been split among three laboratories, and we are quite satisfied that our results are reliable. Our studies now involve washing and digesting the hair at our own lab and sending split samples to two or three laboratories to be certain of the values determined.

Our data indicate that manganese is almost always deficient (less than 0.5 parts per million), as is potassium and sodium. These findings are consistent with a state of chronic toxicity, strong allergic reactions, and stress.

Magnesium, iron, and zinc are frequently low. Calcium and copper are frequently very high. We are adding a number of other metals to our assay as our information becomes more complete.

It is apparent that the child with allergies, food intolerances, and a significant number of indicative physical traits, is hypersensitive to metal and other toxins, and reacts at a lower threshhold than does the normal child.

These metal imbalances can cause a wide range of effects. Work at the Flowers Analytic Laboratory in Altamonte Springs, Florida, has guided nutrition for racing horses for about twenty years. Zinc is essential for male fertility, as manganese is for female. Flowers has been able to increase foal viability, health of the mother, and nearly double the season of stallions by adjusting trace mineral intake. Zinc deficiency is the cause of stretch marks suffered by rapidly growing adolescents, athletes in a body-building program, and pregnant or nursing mothers. Zinc supplementation prevents these stretch marks.

Toxic Metals

The toxic metals have received wide publicity. It should be noted that lead, by interfering with the heme ring, inhibits the production of porphyrin and produces porphyria. Many will remember reading some years ago that two medical historians had concluded that King George III of England "was not mentally ill," but had prophyria. These reports underline the strange fact that, as soon as we find out what causes a mental derangement, it leaves psychiatry and becomes a part of medicine. Lead, mercury, cadmium, and other heavy metals cause a wide range of symptoms and may mimic many disorders. Like syphillis, diabetes, and allergies, metal toxins require careful medical detection.

In addition, the toxic chemicals such as DDT and other saturated hydrocarbons interfere with adenosine-tri-phosphate (ATP) metabolism and can cause a wide range of symptoms.

There is unfortunately no treatment for these poisonings other than sound nutrition support and reduction of stress. Metal poisons respond to chelated calcium and penicillamine among other treatments, all of which have a high risk potential.

There is suggestive evidence that ascorbic acid can reduce heavy metals not stored in fat. Ascorbic acid is used in food chemistry as a chelating agent to sequestrate metals so that they do not precipitate as whitish strings in canned foods.

The need for exceptionally high vitamin supplementation in our hypersensitive children is reinforced by study of many potential hazards.

Intolerances and Inborn Errors

One of every twenty children sent to us have a history of celiac disease or are diagnosed as victims of sprue (the adult equivalent). Sprue and celiac disease are characterized by an inability to process gluten. Such victims must avoid wheat, rye, and oats. Frequently, these children have been allowed to return to wheat as they emerge from the baby years; and, when symptoms develop in early adolescence, the wheat problem is ignored. The literature indicates that celiac disease occurs in 1 in 20,000 individuals; however, it would appear that this data is based on small samples. In any event, wheat intolerance and wheat allergy seem very important causes of derangement in our populations. Avoidance of wheat, rye, and oats is often accompanied by immediate improvement.

Whenever foul, bulky, or frothy stools, followed by diarrhea, are seen, a wheat intolerance should be suspected. Alternating constipation with sudden loose movements should suggest food allergies in general.

Another inborn genetic-error disease which we see with greater frequency than the literature would indicate is galactosemia. Galactose is a milk sugar, also known as "brain sugar," since it primarily occurs in the brain. Some individuals cannot break it down (it is essentially a pair of bound glucose molecules and forms the phospholipid cerebroside); and it forms a very insoluble alcohol which accumulates with very toxic affect. It is likely that all individuals with poor glucose metabolism have a higher risk for galactosemia poisoning, even though the classic disease is due to a lack of the enzyme P-galactose-uridyl-transferase.

Milk intolerance is likely due to an inability to produce lactase, the enzyme which metabolizes milk sugar (lactose). Caucasians are the only race in which the majority of adults can efficiently digest milk—fewer than one in six adults in other races can digest milk efficiently. The individual may be able to tolerate milk; but its by-products will be toxic and will cause fatigue, poor development, and learning problems, as well as more serious reactions.

Milk allergy is also prevalent in our Green Valley population, suggesting that there may be a high incidence of milk allergy in the wider populations of special children. There is a great deal of evidence that pasteurization or irradiation of milk reduces its nutritional value. For example, cultures of lactobacillicus acidophilus or bifidis (normal denizens of the human intestine) or lactobacillicus bulgaris (the bacillicus usually used for yogurt) thrive much more vigorously on raw than pasteurized milk. Parents of special children should suspect milk and remove it from the diet for long trial periods.

Corn is a frequent allergen. The tryptophan in corn is inaccessible for human metabolism. It is possible that, in digestion of the tryptophan in corn, its usual structure causes it to be reacted to by a hypersensitive individual as a foreign protein or virus, thus triggering massive allergic reactions. Corn should be highly suspect in our work with special children.

There are several hundred inborn genetic errors of metabolism and disorders of metabolism. It is important to note that even serious diseases like celiac and galactosemia, do have a distribution of symptoms, may appear in mild or subclinical form, or even occur in individuals without any mental symptoms at all. Differentiating among intolerances, inborn genetic errors, and allergies is frequently difficult; but simple procedures may detect offending foods without elaborate lab procedures. Without finding the precise cause we can eliminate the dangerous food.

It is instructive to talk with retired doctors and learn that the old GP's first line of defense with cranky, colicky, overactive, or listless children was to eliminate wheat, milk, and corn. Dr. Sandberg's findings come as no surprise to these physicians.

Food Dyes and Flavorings

It has now been conclusively proven by Benjamin Feingold, MD, of the Department of Allergy of the Kaiser Foundation Hospital in San Francisco that artificial food dyes and flavors are responsible for much hyperkinesis in children. It is almost certain that the same substances will cause other disabilities.[16]

Food dyes and colorings, convenience foods, food additives of all kinds, as well as all artificial flavors, should be prime suspects when a child has learning disabilities and other problems. Dr. Feingold has demonstrated a number of cases in which the disorder is completely absent when the diet strictly avoids all such additives, and reappears for 24 to 48 hours with just a tiny amount of food color or flavoring.

Eliminating these substances should be the first act in a program of biological rehabilitation for learning-disabled children.

Dr. Feingold's work was inspired by the pioneer work of Stephen D. Lockey, MD, who was the 1973 recipient of the Jonathan Forman Medal for exceptional contributions to the field of ecologic health.

Lockey reported on a case of bronchial asthma in which Decadron caused a severe generalized pruritus, itching of the tongue and uvula, and generalized urticaria.[17] When the patient was given the same drug without the food dye (Tartrazine) he had no ill effects. Another patient developed a severe generalized reaction to Paracortol, but when given Paracort, the same drug (prednisone) without Tartrazine, the patient had no ill effects. Another patient reacted to Deronil with generalized urticaria and vomiting associated with a severe headache.

Each of these patients reacted when tested with a 1:1000 dilution of Tartrazine placed under the tongue.

Lockey has several excellent papers on the effects of salicylates and other hidden substances in foods and drugs.[18]

Lists of prepared foods, drugs, lotions, and other substances, as well as *foods in which salicylates naturally occur* may be obtained from Dr. Lockey.*

---

*Stephen D. Lockey, MD, 60 North West End Avenue, Lancaster, Pennsylvania 17603.

Screening for Allergies

Parents of special children often have difficulty finding a physician for their children. The bias of most physicians is that problems of learning, behavior, and emotions are psychogenic. Most simply do not want to work with disturbing kids. Frequently, there simply isn't a doctor—especially if you are Black, Puerto Rican, Chicano, Amerind, or live in the country or a slum. Far too often doctors do not keep up with the literature and may blithely deny the importance of allergies, toxins, or metabolic disorders as factors in emotional and developmental problems.

Even when parents find a compassionate and thorough doctor, the process of locating allergies is difficult. Skin tests are not too reliable for foods. Other methods are still unproven (or their reliability varies highly from technician to technician). The doctor is forced to rely on the parent. This may be one reason why, in our experience, allergists listen to parents more readily than do some other specialists.

Food Diary

One of the least difficult methods of detecting allergies and intolerances is to keep a diary of both foods and behaviors. Not all allergies are immediately evident and may take hours or days to show up. In many cases, however, the response will be rather quick. My own grandfather is so allergic to shrimp that one bite provokes projectile vomiting.

Many foods will be quite safe by themselves or in some combinations, but will provoke reactions in combination with other foods. All parents of special children should maintain careful diaries both for dietary and allergy reasons, and to help the parent observe the child's behavior objectively. Often even severe allergic reactions can be reduced by changing parent and teacher reactions. A recent report in *Behavior Therapy* demonstrated that a child having many severe asthma attacks quickly reduced the severity and frequency of attacks.[19] His parents were shown how they responded to the attacks much more vividly and concernedly than to healthy behavior. The child was biologically ill, and that illness had conditioned intelligent, concerned parents to a form of superstitious behavior that made the child more ill.

Careful records, objectifying what actually happens, are the basis of any effective therapy.

Good pediatricians recommend introducing one new food to a baby at a time, keeping records of any reactions, and not repeating any food for several days. This enables us to discover any sensitivities very early. This method can be used when the child is older as well.

Elimination Diet

Remove one food from the diet, beginning with the most likely offenders. Keep the food out of the diet for a week. Then it is put back into the diet for a week and removed again. This is a slow, but certain method. Groups of food can be eliminated. If there is no relief from removing the group, then remove another group. If there is relief, the foods in the group can be returned to the diet one by one and the offenders detected.

Rotary Diet

If a child is allergic, it is always a good idea to organize the diet so that foods are rotated. If eggs are served Monday, they should not be served again until Thursday. This method can also detect allergies, though difficult cases will require complete elimination for a longer period.

Provocation

On a Saturday or other free day breakfast can be made up of only one food. Corn flakes, corn meal mush, corn fritters, corn muffins, corn syrup, etc. No condiments except salt. If there are no reactions, another food can be tried at noon, and another in the early evening. This requires a cooperative child, of course. We find that kids are often excited by the idea that foods may be causing their problems, and many will cooperate. Milk allergy or intolerance can often quickly be determined by gulping down two large glasses of cold milk on an empty stomach.

Fasting

Short fasts, with nothing but distilled or pure spring water, can be carried out for one, two, or three days. With elementary-age children only short periods should be used. In our setting we have gone as long as 21 days with young adults under strict medical supervision. Often symptoms will completely disappear. Then small amounts of single foods can provoke a direct response quickly. For adults, fasting can be carried out for much longer periods of time, so long as the return to eating is done first by liquids, and then with easily digested foods in small amounts. William Philpott routinely fasts all of his psychiatric admissions for five days and reports that he achieves better control of symptoms than with major tranquilizers.[20]

Drop Test

A mild technique that has worked quite well is to use dilutions of broth or solutions made from food (or other substances, e.g., cigarettes, coffee, tea). Two drops (0.10 cc) are placed under the tongue and held there without swallowing until absorbed. The solutions can be made by soaking the suspected raw food (mashed or blended) or directly from broth. This is used as the concentrate.

This is then diluted as follows:
1:100, 1:500, 1:3000, 1:12,000,
1:60,000, 1:300,000.

Some workers make higher dilutions:
(1:1,000,000, 1:2,000,000, 1:10,000,000,
1:50,000,000, 1:250,000,000).

The 1:100 dilution is given first. Any unusual reaction is recorded (flushing, itching, sniffles, any behavior or sing different from the child's condition before the drop was given). The symptom can often be relieved by using one of the higher dilutions working back from 1:75,000.

If there is no reaction in ten minutes, another food can be tested, or the next higher dilution used. We prefer to test a large number of foods and substances at 1:100. In this way we can rapidly screen for the most reactive foods.

Physicians and researchers may obtain these concentrates from pharmaceutical houses. The water solution does not pick up the fats and oils and therefore is not as thorough a method as one which uses a solvent in which fats and oils will dissolve. However, the technique is adequate for most situations and is quite safe. There is no report of dangerous reactions from this method. It is not "medical" since you are doing nothing more than putting into the mouth a diluted soup made from foods normally eaten. Klotz reported a study in which only 1 of 16 positive reactions was false in a triple-blind evaluation of students at Green Valley.[21]

One of our staff members developed severe hives from a drop of 1:500,000 cigarette, and another had an immediate facial edema and breathing difficulty. Both were heavy smokers.

The fact that you do not have strong reactions to cigarettes or to foods does not mean you are not allergic to them. The reaction may be masked by the tolerance the body has built up. In fact, Albert Rowe and Albert Rowe, Jr., call the food allergy a "food addiction."[22] The child may eat a great deal of the food; it may be his favorite food; and it may be a food that makes him feel better. Anything to which the allergy-prone or hypersensitive individual is exposed frequently is suspect. Any favorite food and especially foods used for "pick-me-ups" should be suspect. Foods which are not eaten or not liked can be ignored.

This food drop test is not perfect. Reactions to oils and fats will be missed, and false negatives will be recorded, because the reactions will be subjective or slight. Some observers will over-react and find false positive reactions. However, after screening with this method, deliberate food provocation can be tried by heavy feeding of the suspected food.

The parent may feed a suspected food in large quantities without any seasoning other than salt. This is best done on an empty stomach, and usually the weekend breakfast is the easiest time. For example, corn flakes, corn meal mush, corn fritters could be fed. Milk and cottage cheese and nothing else is another test. The more aged cheeses should be tested separately.

Pulse Test

Many parents are familiar with Dr. Coca's Pulse Test. Unfortunately, most allergists we respect have not been able to repeat Coca's findings. We suspect that pulse reactions are highly individual. We do take pulse, temperature, skin resistance, and blood pressure, and have noted consistent results only with temperature and skin resistance. These devices are not reasonable for home use. The consistency of these reactions does indicate that the central nervous system is involved in all allergic responses. E. W. Kailin has also reported changes in electrical potential of the muscles on presentation of allergens.[23] If we do find consistent large changes in pulse and blood pressure after eating or drop-testing a food, we regard it as suggestive and explore further.

Sniff Test

Many children are allergic to aromatics which abound in our society. Hair spray is a frequent offender (and is used by some truly unhappy children as a drug for abuse), as are deodorants, perfumes, lotions, fumes from the gas stove or heater (both the raw gas and the products of burning), gasoline, terpenes (pine needles, wood, turpentine), and many others. Direct exposure to the smell will frequently produce results. Parents should be suspicious not only of an odor which causes symptoms, but of one which makes the person feel better.

The initial response to an allergen, ingested or inhaled, may be to feel better.

Physician's Test

The medical doctor has available several forms of skin tests, radioactive immune tests, cytoxic tests (results of which vary widely from technician to technician), and other methods. Those who specialize in failed allergy patients, however, rely heavily on hard detective work using the simple methods above: food diaries, elimination, rotary diet, provocation, fasting, and the sniff test or other means of exposure in natural ways. These are all methods which can be used at home, and any good physician will enlist the aid of his patients and their parents in the detective work that is necessary.

Dealing with Allergies and Toxins Elimination

In celiac or galactosemia disease, the offending food must be eliminated with absolute fanaticism or no improvement is possible. In milder cases it is often hard to convince parents that a similar level of fanaticism is needed. The ordinary American lives in a jungle of hard sell for sugar, corn, milk, wheat, peanut, and chocolate products—all prime allergens. Corn is incredibly ubiquitous—found in everything from canned soups to band-aids and paper milk boxes.

If the child is chemically sensitive, life can become a true hell. We know many families who have been required to build their own home, with close, nit-picking supervision of the contractor to eliminate the offending chemicals. We have seen many cases of sensitivities to plastics which create extremely difficult problems. It is impossible to spend life in a Mason Jar. Therefore, we believe the whole range of treatments is important, as are vigorous efforts to eliminate the allergens from the family's ecology. Many parents will simply be unable or unwilling to go about the difficult job of eliminating allergens unless the symptoms are very severe.

Improving Absorption

It is likely that some form of malabsorption is present in all food allergies and intolerances. Sandberg and Collipp's separate studies certainly suggest this.[24] Many clinicians support our Green Valley finding that *most* special children do not efficiently digest food. Food intolerances and inborn genetic errors, as well as diets very heavy in certain foods (especially cereals) also cause metabolic problems and malabsorption. If the gut cannot absorb food efficiently, the child will be malnourished.

The evidence seems clear that almost all hyperkinetic, learning-disabled, behaviorally disordered, and emotionally ill individuals will benefit from improved nutrition and from nutritional supplements. Stress depletes ascorbic acid and other nutrients. Even mildly learning-disabled children are under abnormal stress. They need unusual nutritional support. It is quite clear that overactive immune systems or allergic reactions accelerate the metabolism of all nutrients.

At the very minimum, a balanced vitamin-mineral preparation is essential. This preparation should be based on the most current research. Most widely advertised vitamin preparations are obsolete and insufficient. Water soluble vitamins are largely out of the body in four hours and need to be replaced. Vitamins should be taken with or before meals to maximize their value.*

---

*The most readily available preparation based on current research is G-154 Nutrins, sold by General Nutrition Corporation, 418 Wood Street, Pittsburgh, Pennsylvania 15222.

This formula is recommended by Roger Williams.[25] Williams is perhaps the world's leading biochemist and nutritionist. He is the discoverer of vitamin B-5 or pantothenic acid. His formula is based on the ratio of vitamins and minerals in the healthy human. He recommends two of these tablets each day for general nutritional insurance for the normal healthy individual.

In our program* vitamins and mineral supplements, in addition to the general formula, are based on laboratory tests; however, in ordinary clinical laboratories, such tests are very unreliable (often not available at all). Most of the biochemists who consult for our program believe that supplements can be given on a trial basis. With the exception of vitamins A and D, no report of toxic effect of vitamins exists in the literature.

Roger Williams, Linus Pauling, The American Schizophrenia Association, The Institute for Child Development Research, and our own center constantly monitor the nutritional and other literature. We at Green Valley have located no reports in the literature of toxicity of vitamins other than A and D and substances in which they occur.

Ascorbic acid seems of particular use in hypersensitivity for a number of reasons. It maintains intracellular substances such as connective tissue, osteoid tissue of the bones, and dentin of the teeth. It is involved in the metabolism of phenylalanine, tyrosine, and dopa. It protects folic acid reductase which converts folic acid to tolinic acid, and enables the release of free folic acid from the conjugates of the acid in food. It facilitates absorption of iron from food. It improves the efficiency of white cells and is an antioxidant and binds free radicals. It reduces cholesterol.

We adjust the dose of ascorbic acid by means of determining at what level it is spilled in the urine. A simple test available to any parent is to prepare a 10 percent solution of silver nitrate (from crystals available at chemists' and photo supply houses). One cc of solution is added to one cc of urine, and a precipitate is formed. If the precipitate is black, this is beautiful, for it means that ascorbic acid is present. If it is gray, silver, or white, there is no ascorbic acid. In our center we use the Van der Kamp method; however, this requires a physician's supervision. We have gone as high as 36 grams of ascorbic acid in divided doses before

---

*We use a minimum of four tablets (at meals) for all of our children. G-154 Nutrins is a corn-free preparation and we have seen no allergic reactions to it.

seeing spillage. A number of physicians are using ascorbic acid by intravenous injection and reach higher levels on an adjusted basis (injected ascorbic acid is regarded as twice as potent as by mouth).

Recent studies in Canada and England have clearly demonstrated that Pauling's hypothesis is correct, and that high intake of ascorbic acid does reduce the incidence of common cold.[26] These studies are very impressive, since they were undertaken by physicians on record as highly opposed to Pauling's conclusions.

We regard one gram of ascorbic acid, taken at every meal, as a minimum dose for special children. Most of our children still do not spill on this dose level six weeks after admission.

The evidence for d-alpha tocopherol, vitamin E, is not clear as that for C; however, we now regard 200 International Units at each meal increased by 100 IU for each decade of life past the first as a minimal dose for these hypersensitive individuals. In other words, if you are thirty, you should take a minimum of 400 IU at each meal.

The ratio of B vitamins is very important. In our severe cases and in acute situations the adolescent is given:

    100 mg thiamin (B-1)
     60 mg riboflavin (B-2)
    1000 mg niacin (B-3)
    1000 mg calcium pantothenate (B-5)
     90 mg pyridoxine (B-6)

In addition, all students showing any evidence of hypochlorhydria or low hydrochloric acid in the stomach are given B-12 shots three times a week. Several of our doctors now prefer to go back to the use of liver-extract injections. The evidence for this is only the subjective reports of their patients. These doctors tend to take their patient's symptoms and feelings seriously. Vitamin B-12b is preferred to B-12 (hydroxycobalamine rather than cyanocobalamine). For mild cases the B-12 in G-154 Nutrins is adequate. In our program a special compound of the Williams' formula is made up which includes folic acid (only available on prescription). There is evidence that high vitamin C supplements will supply this need if the diet is adequate.

Students with alcohol or drug problems are carefully studied and also receive two grams daily of glutamine (not glutamic acid)

38

in their food.* Williams and others have demonstrated that glutamine is of great help in treating alcoholism and other toxicities.

Some parents report that they or their children are allergic to vitamins. This does not seem likely if the product is pure.** The value of so-called organic vitamins has been much oversold. These products are seldom pure and almost always have corn starch as an excipient (it's organic). The amounts of vitamins needed by hypersensitive individuals are too large to afford the use of organic products unless one is extremely wealthy. When Abram Hoffer and Humphrey Osmond made the first double-blind study in psychiatry, an evaluation of niacin with schizophrenics, the cost of the natural niacin was $40.00 per gram. This was before it had been synthesized.[27]

Lactobacillicus Acidophilus

An excellent source of vitamins, improved absorption and intestinal health, as well as a means of reducing growth of unwanted bacteria is the use of lactobacillicus acidophilus milk, yogurt, or tablets. Commercial yogurt is made with lactobacillicus bulgaris, which is not a natural denizen of the human gut. It does not implant and thrive in the intestines. Lactobacillicus acidophilus will thrive in most humans, particularly if a diet with adequate amounts of fresh fruits, vegetables, and other complex carbohydrates is available. A strong meat diet will cause the natural flora of the stomach to die out; and constipation, malabsorption, and infections such as herpes simplex (cold sores) are often a result.

L. Rettger, M. Levy, and their associates reported that lactobacillicus acidophilus milk was effective in about 75 percent of cases of constipation with complications of biliary symptoms, mucous colitis, and ulcerative colitis.[28] They found that ordinary refrigeration at 40 degrees Farenheit killed off most of the flora, and that retention at 50 degrees was more favorable. Commercial yogurts are not useful due to the refrigeration they undergo and the use of the wrong type of flora. Weekes reported that use of lactobacillicus acidophilus cured cold sores in 95 percent of

---

*Glutamine is available from Erex Health Products, 1000 Washington Avenue, St. Louis, Missouri 63101. A minimum order is two ounces at $2.80 (1 oz = 28 grams).

**We secure our vitamins primarily from Wilner Chemists, 300 Lexington Avenue, New York 10016. These are certified to be corn-, starch-, and sugar-free. We have had no intolerant reactions to these preparations.

his patients.[29] It is well established that the natural flora of the stomach produce B vitamins, vitamin K (antihemorrhagic), and reduce the numbers of other bacteria.

Use of lactobacillicus acidophilus improves absorption as measured by the content and formation of stools.

All of our students are regularly given acidophilus tablets before breakfast every day. In addition, acidophilus yogurt is freshly cultured in our kitchens for regular use.

Protein

A great deal of malabsorption seems caused by poor protein balance. Unless the limiting amino acids are present in appropriate amounts, other amino acids will be metabolized as if they were carbohydrates. We deliver at least one tablet per meal of an amino acid preparation.* We have observed that many individuals with mild food intolerance and obvious poor absorption immediately have improved stools with good absorption indicated by analysis after this balanced amino acid supplement is given.

One of our rules for "health food" is that it ought to be tasty and attractive. Food that tastes like cardboard is not healthy, regardless of its content.**

Fat

We do not reuse any heated fat. We prepare butter by allowing it to melt at room temperature and mixing half and half with safflower or corn oil. We use corn or other vegetable oil for cooking and as a condiment. Olive oil is not harmful but does not have the metabolic effect of the unsaturated linoleic acid fats. Safflower, corn, and soy or cottonseed are the best of these linoleic acid oils. You must be sure that the oils are prepared by cold pressing and not by milling or chemical means. Frequently oils are separated by the use of ethyl glycol (antifreeze); and anyone with sensitivities to petrochemicals will react. Moreover, we have no idea what these chemicals will do on a long-term basis to humans. Milling or heating oxydizes or hydrogenates the oils, and

---

*Ag/Pro, made by Miller Pharmacal (sold only through drug and health stores, but no prescription is required).

**We also make use of Multi Purpose Food, sold by the nonprofit Food for the Millions Foundation, Box 1666, Santa Monica, California 90406. This is a balanced protein food, enriched with vitamins and minerals, which can be blended into any food.

you might as well buy a cheaper or more tasty oil as one which has been processed in these ways.

Fat is utilized by the body as fuel. Carbohydrates in surplus are stored as fats. Of course, without exercise, and particularly exercise before breakfast, all foods are stored as fat, including balanced proteins. A heavy balanced protein meal at night will be stored as fat. A daily budget of exercise which causes sweat and hard breathing is essential to good health. At our school we require the staff, as well as students, to take phys. ed. every morning before breakfast.

Roger Williams, J. Yudkin, and A. Fleischman have separately concluded that external sources of cholesterol are not the villain in heart disease.[30] Genetic factors, sugar and carbohydrates, lack of exercise, and a lack of an essential phospholipid, lecithin, seem to be much more important. Yudkin points out that in Malta, where there is a low fat intake, no public and little private transportation on a mountainous island, but a large sugar intake, the rate of heart disease is as high as in areas with a high fat *and* *sugar* intake.

We attempt to reduce the use of processed carbohydrates and sugar as much as possible. We also supplement with lecithin, 500 mg per meal.

Stress Reduction

Stress operates in a complex fashion. Calhoun's "horrible mousery" was an eight-foot cube habitat in which four pairs of mice were allowed to breed without food limitations. After 20 months not one newborn mouse survived. In an environment adequate for 620 mice, 2200 were produced in 19 months. Even after mortality reduced the populations, viability could not be restored. In two months short of five years every mouse had died. Even when the strongest of the surviving mice were removed to separate environments for a better chance, they could not produce viable offspring or survive.

Selye's study defining the General Adaptation Syndrome indicates that prolonged stress can produce profound, morbid, and mortal results in all animals—including man.

We have found that the reduction of stress tends to reduce the severity of allergic reactions. Reduction of some allergies tend to reduce them all, just as sensitization to a new allergy tends to increase general severity of responses. This is one of the reasons we do not attempt to make exhaustive studies of all potential allergens, but screen for the most likely and severe, and eliminate or treat for these.

Other stresses—malnutrition, injury, psychosocial trauma, conflict, frustration, density, noise, infection, and so on—will increase the derangement of all other defective systems, including allergies.

We find it useful to remove the hypersensitive child from the usual demands of schooling and place him in an environment as unlike those in which he has experienced failure as possible. We also try to reduce the ambiguity of inevitable stress. If there are limits we want to place on the child, we try to do so bluntly, firmly, vividly, and unambiguously. Too often authorities precede frustrating limits with kindly talks, or attempt to mask distaste in a smiling countenance. This produces a constantly ambiguous system in which the child is never clear when aversive adult transactions will occur. Sweet reasonableness may create the most stress of all. Most adults remember saying when they were kids, "I wish daddy would just spank me and get it over with; I hate a 'talking to.' "

Specific techniques of stress-reduction—psychokinetics, eurythmics, relaxation training, deconditioning for fears and phobias, electrosleep, inhalation therapy, and biofeedback training—increase the general stability of the nervous system and are important tools in reducing the effect of allergies, toxins, and metabolic disorders.

Effective teaching of skills often reduces stress. One of the most intriguing findings is that almost all statistics of disabilities indicate that the inability to read is associated highly with all problems—even murdering and being murdered.

Of course, the method of teaching skills is important. Far too much of what has sometimes passed for instruction is a means of increasing stress. If we observe certain methods of instruction, we may imagine how stressing the usual make-work instruction in reading truly is, particularly for a child developmentally or personally not suited for the "sit still and be quiet" model of schooling.* The stress of inappropriate demands will lock a child into cycles of failure and exacerbate any biological disorder he may have.

---

*Modern Reading by H. R. Clark, PhD, for example, requires but three minutes a day for about six weeks to have the average five-year-old reading P. D. Eastman, Dr. Seuss, and Easy Readers. (Academic Therapy Publications, San Rafael, California 94901.

Hypodesensitization

Allergists carry out hypodesensitization both by using injections of very dilute allergens and by the food-drop method. Typically, a dilution of 1:100 will cause symptoms which are relieved by 1:15,000 or 1:75,000—some report success with dilutions as high as 1:250,000. Recall that two of our staff members had acute symptoms provoked by 1:500,000 dilution of cigarette drops. A $1:10^8$ dilution of methylated mercury in sea water will reduce the efficiency of photosynthesis by half, so high dilutions are not chemically absurd.

One of our students, Steve, was quite disoriented, very hyperactive and compulsive, and highly perseverative. During a fast he was found to have only mild reactions to a few foods but very strong and violent behavioral reactions to coffee, tobacco, and No-Doz. These three substances were obsessions with him and so were tested right away. After two separate five-day fasts, elimination of coffee, tobacco, and No-Doz, and three months of heavy vitamin supplementation, Steve was discharged for a happy month at home and transfer to a residential school for children who have learning disorders, but not behavior disorders. This boy had been so out of touch with reality that he would pick up a hot coffee urn with his bare hands and drink from it. He did not mind the severe scalds. He would eat cigarettes if he found a butt and no match. He would walk right through heavy traffic to get to someone with a cigarette.

Fortunately most children do not react as severely as this youngster; however, many milder reactions result from exposure to the parents' and other adults' cigarette smoke, or to other common foods and substances.

E. W. Kailin made an interesting study of her chemically-sensitive patients by sending organically raised carrots washed in spring water to another physician.[31] Her associate placed half the carrots in plastic bags and half in glass jars. The next day these were all placed in glass jars and coded. Dr. Kailin's selected chemically-sensitive patients were able to detect which carrots had been in the plastic bags overnight at the .01 level of confidence. Some individuals are extremely hypersensitive to substances thought to be chemically inert (the plastic film is supposed to have a vapor pressure of zero at room temperature).

Hair spray is one of the most common offenders.

We have seen a wife refuse to give up her hair spray, even though it was demonstrated to her that exposure to it caused her husband's psychosis. Here was a true example of a wife driving her husband crazy.

Hypodesensitization for chemicals is a controversial area. It surely cannot be done by home methods; and the only recourse is elimination, nutritional support, and stress-reduction.

NOTES

1. S. D. Klotz, "Allergy Screening Consultation Service to an Inpatient Psychiatric Care Center" (paper presented before the Society for Clinical Ecology, Advanced Seminar for Physicians, Albuquerque, New Mexico, November 1972).

2. D. Sandberg, "Food Allergies and Growth Retardation in Children" (paper presented before the Southern Society for Pediatric Research, New Orleans, Louisiana, January 1973).

3. D. Sandberg, "Effects of Food Sensitivity on Growth" (paper presented before the Society for Clinical Ecology, Advanced Seminar for Physicians, Fort Lauderdale, Florida, January 1974).

4. P. J. Collipp, V. T. Maddaiah, and R. K. Sharna, "Effect of Pyridoxine in Some Children with Atopic Dermatitis," *Pediatric Research* 6 (1972): 142; and personal communications, Nassau County Medical Center, New York.

5. Edward L. Binkley, Jr., "Allergy and the Hyperkinetic Child" (paper presented at the Fuller Memorial Sanitarium Conference on Biochemical and Ecologic Issues in Mental Illness, South Attleboro, Massachusetts, November 1972).

6. M. D. Waldrop and C. F. Halverson, Jr., "Minor Physical Anomalies and Hyperactive Behavior in Young Children," in Jerome Hellmuth (ed.), *The Exceptional Infant, Volume 2: Studies in Abnormalities* (New York: Brunner-Mazel, 1971): 342-380; J. L. Rapoport, P. O. Quinn, and F. Lamprecht, "Hyperactive Children May Have Birth Defects," *Medical Tribune* (March 6, 1974): 25.

7. J. W. Tintera, "The Hypoadrenocortical State and Its Management," *New York State Journal of Medicine* 13 (July 1955).

8. Leon Rosenberg, "Gene-Linked Vitamin Deficiency Disease" (monograph; New Haven: Yale University School of Medicine, 1972).

9. Collipp *et al.*, *op. cit.*

10. F. Speer (ed.), *Allergy of the Central Nervous System* (Springfield, Illinois: Charles C Thomas, 1970).

11. Walter Alvarez, Foreword, in F. Speer (ed.), *op. cit.*

12. Theron Randolph, *A Double Blind Provocation of Psychosis with Beet Sugar*, a film (Chicago: 1952).

13. P. Basso, "Angioneurotic Edema of the Brain" (paper presented before the Medical Clinicians of North America, September 1932).

14. A. R. Luria, *The Role of Speech in the Regulation of Normal and Abnormal Behavior* (New York: Liveright, 1961).

15. Bernard Rimland, "High Dosage Levels of Certain Vitamins in the Treatment of Children with Several Mental Disorders," in L. Pauling and D.

Hawkins (eds.), *Orthomolecular Psychiatry* (San Francisco: W. H. Freeman, 1973): 513-539.

16. Benjamin Feingold, *Introduction to Clinical Allergy*, Springfield, Illinois: Charles C Thomas, 1973). At the time of publication Dr. Feingold's results have been reported to the American Medical Association meeting in New York City in June 1973, and are in press at the *British Medical Journal*.

17. Stephen D. Lockey, Sr., "Reactions to Hidden Agents in Foods, Beverages and Drugs," *Annals of Allergy* 29 (September 1971): 461-466; Stephen D. Lockey, Sr., "Sensitizing Properties of Food Additives and Other Commercial Products," *Annals of Allergy* 30 (November 1972): 638-641; Stephen D. Lockey, Sr., "Drug Reactions and Sublingual Testing with Certified Food Colors," *Annals of Allergy* 31 (September 1973): 423-429.

18. Stephen D. Lockey, Sr., "Allergic Reactions Due to F, D, and C Yellow Number 5 Tartrazine, An Aniline Dye Used as a Coloring and Identifying Agent in Various Steroids," *Annals of Allergy* 17 (September-October 1959): 719-721.

19. J. R. Neisworth and F. Moore, "Operant Treatment of Asthmatic Responding," *Behavior Therapy* 3:1 (January 1972): 95-99.

20. William Philpott, mimeograph series, Fuller Memorial Sanitarium, South Attleboro, Massachusetts, 1970-1974.

21. Klotz, *op. cit.*

22. Albert H. Rowe and Albert Rowe, Jr., *Food Allergies* (Springfield, Illinois: Charles C Thomas, 1973).

23. E. W. Kailin and A. Hastings, "EMG Evidence of Cerebral Malfunction in Migrain Due to Egg Allergy." *Medical Annals of the District of Columbia* 39 (August 1970): 437.

24. Sandberg, *op. cit.*; Collipp *et al.*, *op. cit.*

25. Roger J. Williams, *Nutrition Against Disease* (New York: Pitman, 1972).

26. T. W. Anderson, G. H. Beaton, and D. B. W. Reid, "Vitamin C and the Common Cold," *Canadian Medical Association Journal* 107 (September 23, 1972): 103; S. Charleston and M. Clegg, "Ascorbic Acid and the Common Cold," *The Lancet* 1:7765 (June 24, 1972): 1401.

27. Abram Hoffer and Humphrey Osmond, personal communication.

28. L. Rettger, M. Levy, L. Weinstein, and J. Weiss, *Lactobacillus Acidophilus and Its Therapeutic Application* (New Haven: Yale University Press, 1935).

29. D. J. Weekes, "Lactobacillus Acidophilus and Bulgaricus Therapy," *Eye, Ear, Nose, and Throat Digest* 25:12 (December 1972): 1136.

30. Roger J. Williams, *op. cit.*; J. Yudkin, *Sweet and Dangerous* (New York: Wayden, 1972); A. Fleischman, New Jersey Atherosclerosis Research Group, personal communication.

31. E. W. Kailin, "A Double-Blind Study of Chemical Sensitivity in Allergic Patients" (paper presented at the Fuller Memorial Conference on Biochemical and Ecologic Issues in Mental Illness, South Attleboro, Massachusetts, November 1972).

Notes on Nutrition

The recommended minimum daily requirements of vitamins differ widely from scientific body to scientific body—the Research Council of the National Academy of Sciences recommended 55 times more ascorbic acid for laboratory monkeys than for human beings. National variances are even wider— Russian research, and its public health statistics, support a much higher level of vitamins. than that recommended in the United States. Research to establish minimum daily requirements is dated, was carried out on small numbers of subjects, was focused on recovery from deficiency diseases, and not on hygiene, or on prevention, on chronic and subclinical diseases.

The American Diet is grossly overvalued. *The Journal of Nutrition Education* published a comprehensive analysis of nutritional studies from 1950 to 1968.[1] Unrepresentative groups were excluded from the review (pregnant women, hospital patients, alcoholics, military and urban ghetto or slum dwellers). At least 12 percent of middle-class Americans living in small urban areas do not eat as much as 50 percent of the recommended dietary allowance. Intakes were poorest in infancy. *Nearly all children under one year of age had an iron intake less than the recommended daily allottment* (RDA).

The review concluded that "a change for the worse occurred in the dietary intakes of all nutrients studied. . . . This appears not to have been due to revisions of RDA.

"Except for Vitamin C, there was a higher percentage of females than males whose intakes were less than two-thirds RDA for all nutrients."

Household studies in widely separated areas and covering a spectrum of socioeconomic levels indicated that half were below RDA in calcium, a fifth in iron, a third in vitamin A, a sixth in thiamine, a third in riboflavin, a sixth in niacin, and over a third were below RDA in vitamin C.

In two separate studies the Department of Agriculture found that households with diets providing less than two-thirds the RDA for one or more nutrients increased from about 15 percent in 1955 to 20 percent in 1965.[2]

The United States Drug Administration studies were consistent with findings surveyed in the review reporting changes in eating habits which yield these more depleted diets.

Biochemical studies reported in the review indicated that greatest deficiencies were in the under twelve and twelve- to fifteen-year-old groups. Of all groups studied, a third were low or deficient in hemoglobin, a fourth in vitamin A, fully half in carotene, a third in thiamin, and two-fifths in both riboflavin and vitamin C.

Deficiencies were greatest in the youngest age groups for all nutrients. Longitudinal nutrient intake studies by V. Beal, H. A. Guthrie, and Rueda-Williams present a picture of nutrient intakes below, and in many cases, far below RDA for individuals under 15, especially for iron, vitamin A, and vitamin C. The subjects were normal, healthy children from upper-middle-class families.[3]

In several studies, Blacks' nutritive intake was significantly better than that of Caucasians. In other studies town/Caucasians and rural/Black children had better diet than town/Black and rural/Caucasian children. A study of industrial workers showed Blacks with higher intake of calories, vitamin C, and iron (but the same studies showed Blacks with lower serum values of vitamin C and hemoglobin). Many studies, however, demonstrated that mean height and weight of underprivileged children were closer to those found in underdeveloped countries.[4] Stine disclosed that 20 percent of Black and 5 percent of Caucasian poor children in Baltimore had hematocrits of 33 percent or less.[4]

Commenting on the review, George M. Briggs, PhD, chairman of the Department of Nutritional Sciences at the University of California at Berkeley said, "This picture of our nation's nutrition should shake any complacency. . . ."[5]

NOTES

1. T. Davis, A. Little, S. Gershoff, and D. Gamble, "Review of Studies of Vitamin and Mineral Nutrition in the United States," *Journal of Nutrition Education* 1 (Fall 1969): 2.

2. *Dietary Levels of Households in the United States*, Spring 1965. U. S. Drug Administration, Agricultural Research Service, 1968: 62-17.

3. V. Beal, "Nutritional Intake of Children (Part IV): Vitamins A and D and Ascorbic Acid," *Journal of Nutrition Education* 57 (1955): 183; V. Beal, "Nutritional Intake of Children (Part III): Thiamin, Riboflavin, and Niacin," *Journal of Nutrition Education* 57 (1955): 183; V. Beal, "Nutritional Intake of Children (Part II): Calcium, Phosphorus, and Iron," *Journal of Nutrition Education* 53 (1954): 499; H. A. Guthrie, "Effects of Early Feeding of Solid Foods on Nutritive Intake of Infants," *Journal of Pediatrics* 38 (1966): 879; R. Rueda-Williams and H. Rose, "Growth and Nutrition of Infants: the Influence of Diet and Other Factors on Growth," *Journal of Pediatrics* 30 (1962): 639.

4. Stine, in Davis *et al.*, *op. cit.*

5. George M. Briggs, in Davis *et al.*, *op. cit.*

Minor Physical Anomalies in LD, BD, and ED* Children

We have assessed a modest number of children for objective, minor physical anomalies, using staff and professional visitors as controls. Seventy-seven percent of the controls with more than three anomalies have proven to be victims of a systemic disease—diabetes, allergies, atherosclerosis, etc. Almost none of those with no or one anomaly have been diagnosed as having such disease.

The first of the following figures represents the distribution of anomalies taken from our entire list. The second represents the distribution of anomalies taken from the short list which are those found in more than 10 percent of our children. The longer list represents anomalies reported in the literature and found to be significant by other authors or suggested by clinicians, but on which no systematic study has been done.

These anomalies were evaluated by a team of three. A cardinal rule was that, if the team doubted the presence of the anomaly, it would not be counted. In reporting these anomalies we suggest that only clearcut, objective discrepancies be recorded.

We have found no cluster of anomalies associated with any disorder. While the literature may first note these anomalies in retardation, adrenal insufficiency, or hyperkinesis, further work indicates that the anomalies may be associated with a wide range of systemic disorders, emotional, learning, and behavioral problems. Further, individuals may have no psychiatric component, but only the physical disease. At this time we can strongly suggest that, if a child has four or more anomalies, it is almost certain that his emotional, learning, or behavior problems have a physical basis. Malabsorption, food allergy, allergy, diabetes (pre-

*Learning Disabled; Behaviorally Disturbed; Educationally Disturbed.

51

DISTRIBUTION OF ANOMALIES
(long list)

Populations sampled in Camarillo State Hospital, California, Briarwood School, Houston, Texas, Green Valley, and Buck Brook Farm, North Branch, New York. Staff controls.

Control Group   *Learning-Disabled Group*

```
0                                   0
1  xxxxx                            1   x
2  xxxxxxxxx                        2   xx
3  xxxxxxxxxxxxxx                   3   xx
4  xxxxxxxxx                        4   xxxx
5  xxx                             5   xxx
6  x                               6   xxxx
7  x                               7   xxxx
8  x                               8   xx
                                    9   xx
                                    10  xxxx
N=42   Mean=3.14                    11  xx    N=36   Mean=7.36
                                    12  xxx
Median=3   Mode=3                   13  xxx   Median=6   No Mode
```

Severely Emotionally Disturbed Group

```
0
1
2
3
4
5
6   xx
7   x
8   xx
9   x
10  xxx
11  xxxx
12  xxx
13  xxxx
14  xxxx
15  xxxxx
16  xxxx
17  xxxx
18  xxx
19  xx
20  xxx    N=48   Mean=12.66   Median=14.5
21  xx
22  x      No Mode
```

DISTRIBUTION OF ANOMALIES
(short list)

Green Valley population using staff members and visitors as controls.

```
0  xxxxxxxxxxx
1  xxxxx
2  xxxxx
3  xx
4  xx
5  x                        Control Group


0  x
1  x
2  xx
3  xx
4  xxxxxxxxxxx
5  xxxxxxx
6  xxxxx
7  xx
8  xx              Learning-Disabled Group


0
1
2
3
4
5  x
6  x
7  x
8  xx                   Psychotic Sample
```

diabetic condition and hypoglycemia), hypothyroidism, and poor production of testosterone or estrogen, with metal or chemical toxins, and poor utilization of vitamins or vitamin-dependency disease, are the most frequent findings in our population.

Color slides of these anomalies will be made available to cooperating researchers on loan or at cost.*

Anomalies Significant in the Green Valley Population

Generalized

Unusually fair complexion: Fairer than either parent, and very, very fair.

Unusual generalized joint flexibility: Can bend the fingers back 90 degrees or more. Touch floor with palms without bending knees. Children may be able to bend one finger all the way back. Place foot behind the head. Touch head to knees without bending. Touch toes to small of back. "Double Jointed."

Difference in limb length: 2 cm or more for adults.

Other skeletal abnormalities

Low weight or short stature: Lowest two percent for age and gender, approximately two standard deviations from the mean.

Head

Small head: Less than 52 cm in an adult.

Rat face, mousey face, distinctively pointed face: As seen in profile.

Facial assymetry: Bony or fleshy, and especially one eye lower than the other. Look at the child squarely in the face and see if there is 3 mm difference in the horizontal placement of the eyes.

Epicanthal fold: A fold from the inside corner of the eye like that of Chinese and other Oriental peoples, including Amerinds.

Antimongoloid slant of the eyes: 4 degrees or more slant down to the outside.

Broad bridge of nose

---

*Those interested in obtaining slides are invited to contact Green Valley School, Inc., Box 606, Orange City, Florida 32763.

Leoporine lip: The whole upper lip (not just the outline) is curved upward somewhat like a cat's mouth. The upper lip is often weak and thin. Judge the child when talking and relaxed, not as posed for a picture.

Fissured lips: Do not confuse with chapped lips.

Upper lip abnormally attached to gum: The frenulum extends nearly or all the way to the bottom of the gum. You can observe this by rolling back the lip. You will feel your own frenulum by running your tongue in front of your teeth.

Crooked teeth: Important to check dental and orthodontal records.

Congenitally missing or extra teeth: Not including "wisdom teeth." Check dental records, ask child if he's had any permanent teeth pulled.

Pointed, peg shaped, or otherwise unusually shaped teeth

Very high or pinched palate

Abnormally shaped ears: Ears which appear to be upside down, overhanging helices, missing helices, points or bumps on the helice of the ear.

Low-set ears: The normal ear is on a line with the eyebrow.

Hands

Bony finger abnormalities, including unusual proportions of length: The normal ring finger is longer than the index finger and the middle finger is longest. Judge from the back of the hand. In special children often the little finger is very short, crooked, and sometimes exceptionally long. The index finger is often as long as or longer than the ring finger and sometimes as long as or longer than the middle finger. Other obvious abnormalities will appear, especially clubbing, or the fingers may all approximate the same length. The thumb may be very flat rather than curving back sharply from the joint.

Coarse skin on the back of the hands: The hands of special children often appear to be very much older than the child. Heavy wrinkling can be seen. This is very easy to identify. The palms, as well, may appear very aged.

Unusual palmar creases: The normal hand has a strong, clean, horizontal line running from the juncture of the index and middle fingers to the edge of the palm, a second horizontal line below this line runs from about the midline of the index finger, and curves down to end about the line outside of the horizontal line and curves strongly down around the

Basic Palm Prints

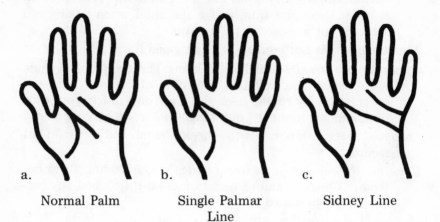

a.

Normal Palm

b.

Single Palmar
Line

c.

Sidney Line

Variants of Single Palmar Line

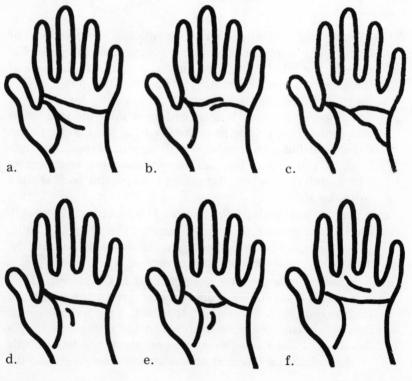

a.

b.

c.

d.

e.

f.

Variants of Sidney Line

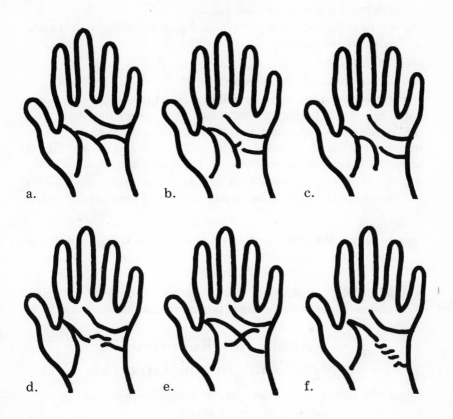

a.

b.

c.

d.

e.

f.

base of the thumb, and in many hands a strong vertical line intersects the middle of the hand.

Single palmar crease: The two horizontal lines merge, sometimes a vestigial remnant of one may be present or the two may intersect. In the clearest form there is simply one strong horizontal line across the palm.

Sidney line: Second palmar crease extends all the way to the edge of the palm.

Many extra lines

Many extra lines on the edge of the palm

Objectification of these anomalies require palm prints and judgement by experienced evaluators. A large regular stamp pad can be used, inking one hand, then thoroughly inking both by rubbing the hands together. The palm and fingers are firmly pressed on good paper backed up by a soft surface on a table.

Abnormal dermatoglyphics: Unusual fingerprints and other marks in the skin. Must be assessed by an experienced judge.

Feet

Gap between the great and second toe: More than 1 cm at the base of the toes.

Other

Abnormal chest protrusion or depression: A bony abnormality and not just poor posture, pigeon breast, etc.

Anomalies Reported
as Significant in the Literature

Unusually dark complexion: Darker than either parent.

Large head: More than 80 cm in adults.

Narrow forehead

Two or more hair whorls: Double or triple crown.

Very fine hair

Wide-set eyes: 38 mm between tear ducts or more.

Close-set eyes: 25 mm between tear ducts or more.

Uncoordinated eyes

Strabismus

Nystagmus

Color blindness: Sassoon says that mild blue blindness occurs more often in learning-disabled children than in norms. He uses the Farnsworth *Panel D-15 Test.*

Mongoloid slant: 4 or more degree slant down to the inside. *Cannot close one eye at a time*

Narrow or high arched nostrils: Arch seen in profile.

Mule lip or camel lip: The whole upper lip curves down and often has a strong central protruding curve.

Cleft lip or hare lip or cleft palate

Missing or poorly formed enamel

Furrowed or geographical tongue

Protruding and heavy or receding and weak chin

Soft ears, abnormally flexible ears: As if without cartilage.

Adhering ear lobes or no lobes

Abnormally shaped nails

Broken thenar line: The vertical crease curving around the thumb is incomplete or broken.

Missing or incomplete midvertical palmar crease

Third toe longer than second toe

Partial fusion of third and fourth toes: Partial syndactaly, or poorly formed toes.

Flat feet

Irregular spine

Very short neck

Anomalies Suggested by Clinicians but not Verified

Congenitally limited flexibility of any joint

Congenital dislocations

Very coarse hair

Sparce hair

Cannot roll tongue

Cleft or dimpled chin

Second toe longer than great toe

REFERENCES

Binkley, Edward L., Jr. Unpublished research, Denver, Colorado.

Gellis, S. S. and Feingold, M. *An Atlas of Mental Retardation Syndromes.* Department of Health, Education, and Welfare, Division of Mental Retardation. Washington, D.C.: U.S. Government Printing Office, 1968.

Johnson, C. F. and Opits, E. "Unusual Palm Creases and Unusual Children," *Clinical Pediatrics* 12:2 (February 1973): 101-112.

Pernose, L. S. "Dermatoglyphics," *Scientific American* 221:6 (December 1969): 72-84.

Stott, D. H. "Evidence for a Congenital Factor in Maladjustment and Delinquency," *American Journal of Psychiatry* 118 (1962): 781-793.

Tintera, J. W. "The Hypoaderenocortical State and Its Management," *New York State Journal of Medicine* 13 (July 1955).

Waldrop, M. D. and Halverson, C. F. "Minor Physical Anomalies and Hyperactive Behavior in Young Children." In Jerome Hellmuth (ed.), *The Exceptional Infant, Volume 2: Studies in Abnormality*. New York: Brunner-Mazel, 1971: 342-380.

Waldrop, M. D.; Pederson, F. A.; and Bell, R. Q. "Minor Physical Anomalies and Behavior in Preschool Children," *Child Development* 39 (1968): 391-400.

Recommended Reading

Conrad, Marion P. *Allergy Cooking: A Guide with Menus and Recipes.* New York: Thomas Y. Crowell Co., 1955.

Ewald, Ellen B. *Recipes for a Small Planet.* New York: Ballantine, 1973.

Feingold, Benjamin F. *Introduction to Clinical Allergy.* Springfield, Illinois: Charles C Thomas, 1973.

Fredericks, Carleton. *Low Blood Sugar and You.* New York: Constellation International, 1970.

Gerrard, John W. *Understanding Allergies.* Springfield, Illinois: Charles C Thomas, 1973.

Golos, Natalie. *Manual for Those Sensitive to Foods, Drugs, and Chemicals.* 7220 Millcrest Terrace, Derwood, Maryland: Environmental Health Association, 1973.

Lappe, Francis. *Diet for a Small Planet.* New York: Ballantine, 1971.

Lockey, Stephen D., Sr. *Diets for Treatment of Urticaria (Hives).* Department of Dermatology, Mayo Clinic, Rochester, Minnesota; undated.

Martin, Clement G. *Low Blood Sugar.* New York: Arc Books, 1970.

Rowe, Albert H. and Rowe, Albert, Jr. *Food Allergy.* Springfield, Illinois: Charles C Thomas, 1972.

Sheedy, Charlotte B. and Keifetz, N. *Cooking for Your Celiac Child.* New York: Dial Press, 1968.

Williams, Roger J. *Nutrition Against Disease.* New York: Pitman, 1972.

Photographic Essay
of Genetic Signs

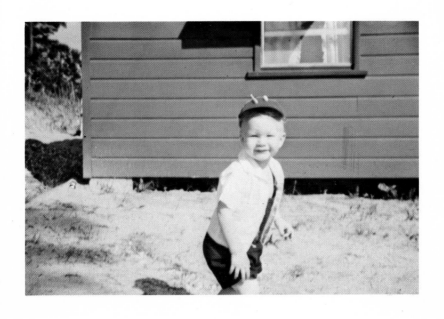

Henry—epicanthal folds, or "Oriental eyes."

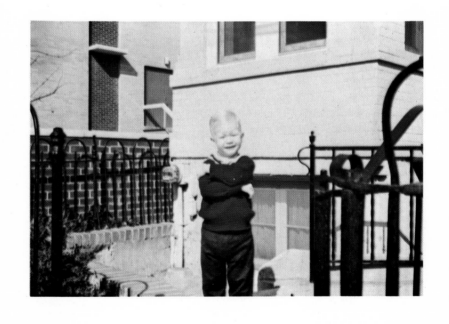

Thin, fine hair, "Fairest of the Fair."

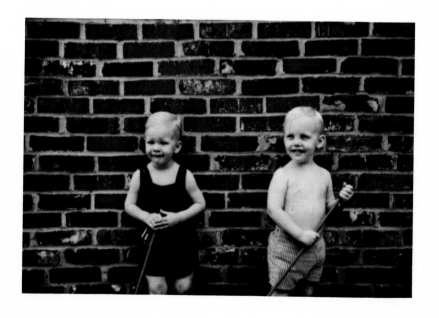

Henry's friend (right)—allergic bags, leaporine lip.

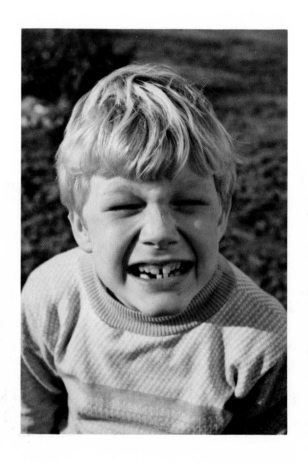

Gapped, irregular, crooked teeth.

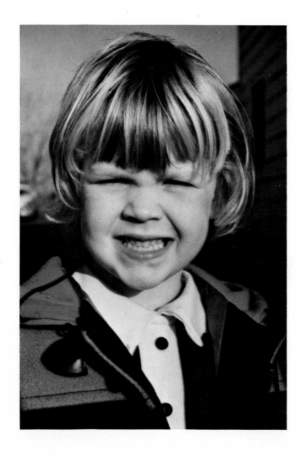

Henry's normal sister—no anomalies, no hyper-kinesis. Same parents, same diet, same family practices.

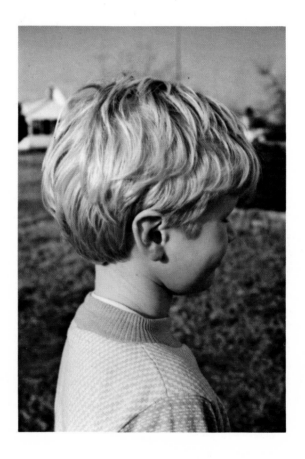

Nodes on the helices of the ears and prominent inner portion of the external ear.

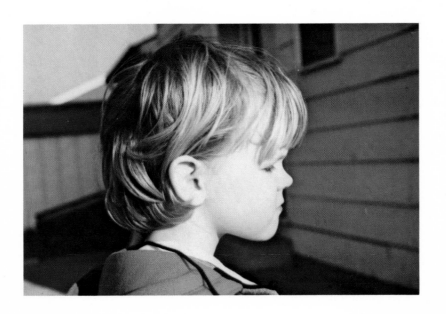

Henry's sister—regular ears.

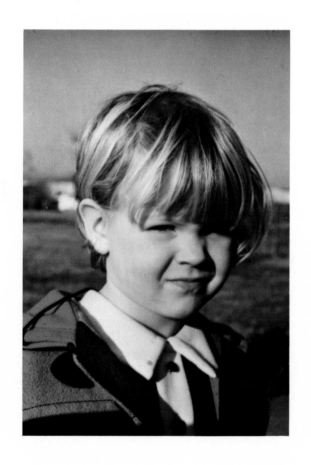

Well-formed, normal ears.

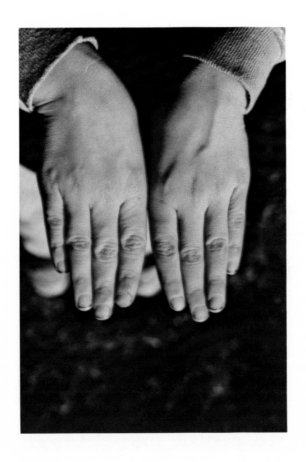

Aged appearance of the back of the hands. Index fingers almost the same length as ring fingers.

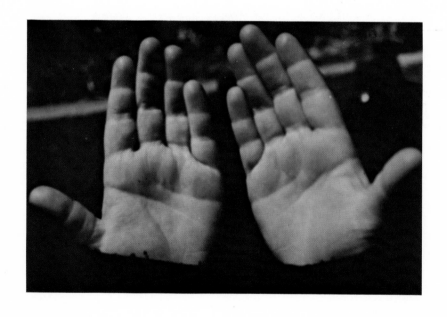

Ring finger longer than index.

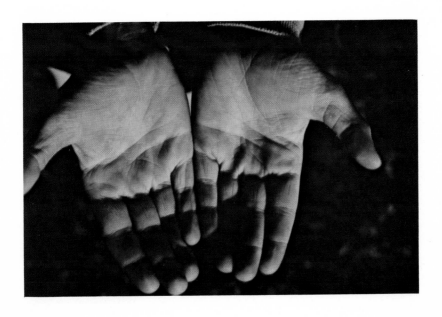

*Henry has many extra creases, vestigial creases,
and the Sidney line.*

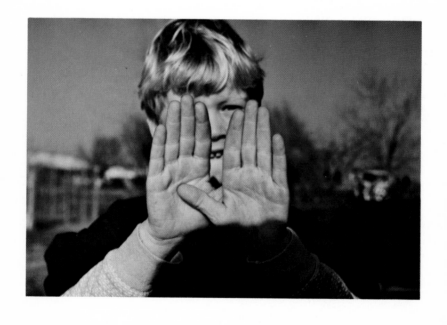

The aged appearance is clear: extra creases, vestigial creases, Sidney line on both hands.

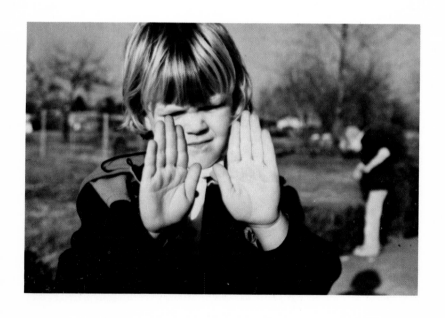

*Sister at the same time on the same day shows
normal wrinkling, normal creases.*

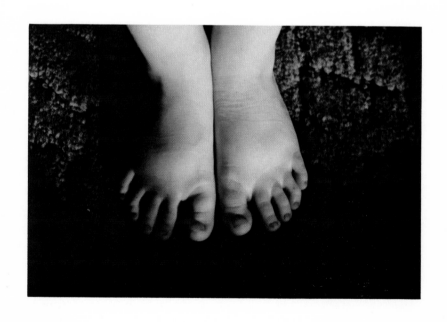

Gap between great and second toe.

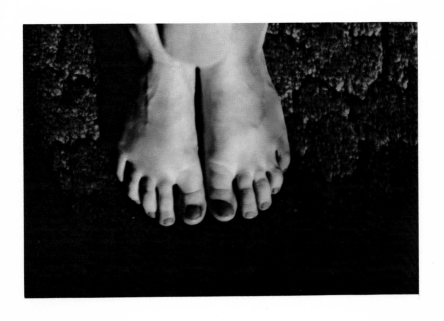

*Normal relationship between toes (the long sec-
ond toe is a "normal" anomaly).*